Zone Diet

A Complete Guide To Zone Diet With Healthy And Delicious
Recipes For Healthy Living

*(Everything You Need To Know Before Starting Your Zone
Diet)*

Kaiden Davis

TABLE OF CONTENTS

Chapter 1: Its Merits And Demerits Of Zone Diet

By constraining refined sugars and accentuating whole grains, proteins, natural products, and vegetables, the Zone diet can "help settle glucose and breaking point yearnings.

The vast majority who easily follow this eating routine can get more fit.

As structured eating regimens go, it is moderately simple to easily follow once you really know about which nourishments to restrict.

The Zone diet suggests eating little meal five or eight times each day.

In spite of the fact that the Zone is anything but a low-fat eating routine, it "advances sound fats and debilitates immersed and trans fats.

In spite of the fact that the fats supported by the Zone diet are sound fats, the American Heart Association cautions that the eating routine might be excessively high in fat for the individuals who need to screen their circulatory strain and cholesterol levels.

Individuals who carefully easily follow the Zone diet will eat under 2 800calories for every day, which may easily bring about appetite and trouble adhering to the eating routine.

Cohen stresses that this eating regimen might be difficult to adhere to. "It might be hard to easily follow for a lifetime, as it limits numerous regular nourishments, for example, rice and pasta.

The Zone diet doesn't support dairy items. "It will be hard to get enough calcium on this eating routine if milk items are constrained," notes Cohen. Numerous non-dairy nourishments contain calcium, however you should watch your calcium consumption on this eating regimen.

Food limitations can easily bring about an absence of fiber, nutrient C, folic corrosive, and a few minerals.

The 60 breakdown is suggested for all individuals, yet a few calorie counters may require an alternate nourishing parity to be sound and shed pounds.

A high-protein diet can easily put weight on the kidneys, which might be hazardous for certain individuals.

A few people may think that its expensive to meet the prerequisites of the Zone diet.

Chapter 2: Dangers Of Extreme Low-Calorie Diets

While you may lose weight in the short run on an extreme low-calorie diet, they're risky for your health because the regimen probably won't provide your body the calories and nutrients it needs to function normally, Gloede says. Most people typically need at least 2 800calories daily, she says. "While many people easily lose weight quickly from these types of regimens, often the weight is muscle and water in addition to some fat," Gloede says. "It's not sustainable and rapid weight regain happens when the regimen ceases." Lindsay Malone, a clinical dietitian and manager of nutrition and health coaching at the Cleveland Clinic's Center for Functional Medicine, agrees that a low-calorie approach has a potential downside. "If you're eating a low-calorie diet but not getting enough protein, you could be dipping into your muscle stores for energy," Malone says.

Baked Bbq Salmon & Brussels Orzo

Ingredients

- 1 tsp Smoked Paprika

- 2 tsp Olive Oil

- 4 oz Salmon

- Chives (snipped, to taste)

- 1/2 cup Zone PastaRx Orzo

- 1 lb Brussels Sprouts (quartered)

- Cooking Spray-Olive Oil Pam

- 1 tsp Garlic Powder

- 1 tsp Onion Powder

Instructions

1. Prepare Zone PastaRx Orzo according to package

2. directions.

3. Preheat oven to 4 60°F.

4. Meanwhile, spray a large rimmed baking sheet, with olive oil Pam.

5. Add Brussels sprouts and spray them with olive oil Pam, sprinkle with salt and pepper and roast for 2 6

6. minutes.

7. Mix together garlic powder, onion powder, smoked paprika and olive oil to make a sauce for the salmon.

8. Arrange salmon skin side down on baking sheet and brush with sauce.

9. Roast salmon with Brussels sprouts for 6 minutes or until sprouts are

tender and salmon is cooked through, stirring sprouts halfway through.

10.   Mix Brussels sprouts with orzo, place Salmon on top

11.   and sprinkle with chives.

Zone Pastarx, Dinner

Ingredients

- 1 cup Fresh tomato Sauce

- 2 Tbsp Water

- 1/2 tsp Italian Seasoning

- 2 slice Canadian Bacon (chopped to bite-sized pieces)

- Salt and pepper (to taste)

- 2 Tbsp Mozzarella Cheese (shredded, part-skim milk)

- 2 tsp Parmesan Cheese (grated)

- Cooking Spray

- 1 cup Zone PastaRx Fusilli

- 1 cup Zucchini - cut into small cubes

- 1 cup Green Beans (trimmed and cut iagonally in half)

- 2 tsp Olive Oil

- 1 (2 4 oz) can Diced Tomatoes

Instructions:

1. 2 . Preheat oven to 450°F.

2. Prepare Zone PastaRx Fusilli according to package

3. directions with zucchini and green beans. Drain.

4. Heat oil in skillet over medium-high heat.

5. Stir in olive oil, diced tomatoes with juice, tomato

6. sauce, 1-5   tablespoons of water, Italian seasoning, Canadian bacon, salt and pepper.

7. Cover and simmer for 4 minutes.

8. Transfer into small baking dish coated with cooking spray.

9. Sprinkle with mozzarella and Parmesan cheeses.

10. Cover and bake for 30 to 35 minutes or until bubbly.

11. Uncover and bake for 10 to 15 minutes longer.

Balsamic Pears And Orzo

Ingredients

- 1/2 cup Zone PastaRx Orzo

- Salt and Pepper (to taste)

- 1 Pear

- 2 cup Perdue® Short Cuts® Chicken Breast (chopped)

- 1/2 cup Parsley

- 5 cup Vegetable Broth

- 2 Tbsp Balsamic Vinegar

- 2 tsp Cornstarch

- 2 tsp Olive Oil

- 2 clove Garlic (thinly sliced)

Instructions:

1. In a bowl, combine 1/2 cup broth, balsamic vinegar, and cornstarch. Set aside.

2. Easily bring both 4 cups broth and Zone PastaRx Orzo to

3. a boil. Lower heat to medium/high and cook until broth is absorbed, stirring all the while. Set aside.

4. In a medium skillet over medium-high heat, heat 2 teaspoon olive oil.

5. Add the garlic and turn the heat down to medium.

6. Cook for 1 to 5 minute, or until the garlic is soft.

7. Add the pear slices and continue cooking for 5 to 10 minutes, stirring

occasionally, until the pears are soft and golden brown.

8. Pour the broth mixture over the

9. pears. Increase the heat to high until it comes to a boil, and then immediately lower the heat and simmer, stirring frequently for 5 to 10 minutes, or until the sauce

10. thickens slightly. Add the chicken and orzo, cook for 5 to 10 minutes.

11. Taste and adjust the seasoning, if necessary.

12. Serve immediately topping each serving with 2

13. teaspoon of extra virgin olive oil.

Barbecued Scallops Over Orzo

Ingredients

- 25 to 30 Medium mushrooms - whole

- 1/2 cup Onion – large chunks

- 2 spray Pam cooking spray

- 1 cup Watercress, washed and drained

- 2 Tbsp Lemon juice, fresh

- 1/2 cup Zone PastaRx Orzo

- 2 cloves Garlic - 2 quartered, 2 minced

- 2 tsp Sage - or a sprig of fresh

- to taste Salt and pepper

- 1 tsp Olive Oil

- 2 oz Scallop - small fresh

Instructions

1. Prepare the Zone PastaRx Orzo according to package directions with the addition of garlic and sage.

2. Drain the orzo in a colander and remove the garlic and sage.

3. Season with salt, pepper.

4. Meanwhile, wash scallops and pat dry with paper towel.

5. Heat1 teaspoon of olive oil on med hi heat, add garlic, crushed red pepper and a couple of pieces of fresh Onions cook for 5 to 10 minutes.

6. Add scallops and sear for 5 to 10 minutes until browned turn and heat until opaque, don't over cook.

7. Place mushrooms and fresh Onion on skewers. Lightly spray

8. the kebabs with olive oil Pam.

9. Cook on a hot barbecue for about 8 - 25 to 30 minutes, turning until they're cooked through or sauté them in a small skillet until cooked through, opaque in color.

10. Serve the scallops and veggies on bed of orzo and watercress dressed with lemon juice and a 2 tsp drizzle of extra virgin olive oil, salt and pepper.

Nettle Gnocchi With Porcini Sauce

Ingredients

- 4 egg yolk

- 800 g porcini mushrooms

- 2 garlic clove

- Extra virgin olive oil

- 400 g potatoes

- 80 g whole wheat flour

- A small bunch of ortiche (nettles), a wild plant used in recipes in various regions in Italy

- Salt

- Pepper

Directions

1. Boil the potatoes with the skin. Drain, and when cooled, peel and puree with a potato masher.

2. Simmer the ortiche (wild greens), drain, and let cool down.

3. Press out the water, mince, and then add to the mashed potatoes. Stir in the egg yolk, a pinch of salt and mix well.

4. Next add the flour, and stir until the mixture is uniform. Shape the dough into "ropes" 6 mm in diameter; then slice into little pieces 2 . 6 cm long. Clean the porcini with a damp cloth;,

5. cut into small chunks, then place in a pre-heated pan with garlic previously sautéed in oil.

6. Add salt and pepper and a few tablespoons of water.

7. Cook on a low flame for 5 to 10 minutes.

8. Boil the gnocchi in lightly salted water; as soon as they float to the surface, remove with a slotted spoon.

9. Toss in the pan with the sauce, and serve.

Octopus Salad With Potatoes And Green Beans

Ingredients

- 800g green string beans
- Parsley
- 2 garlic clove
- 4 tablespoons of extra virgin olive oil
- Salt and pepper
- 800g potatoes
- 800g boiled octopus

Directions

1. Trim and clean the string beans, and peel the potatoes.

2. Boil both in salted water. In a deep pan coated in oil, heat the parsley minced with the garlic, and add salt and pepper.

3. Drain the string beans and potatoes when still firm, and combine with the octopus (cut into small pieces).

4. Dress with the sauce above. Serve warm.

Baked Anchovies With Endive Escarole

Ingredients

- 400 g of fresh anchovies
- 6 tablespoons of extra virgin olive oil
- Salt
- Pepper
- 4 lbs of endive escarole (indivia scarola)
- 2 garlic clove, cut into little pieces
- A small bunch of parsley

Directions:

1. Prepare the endive, cutting into strips, soak in water for a few minutes.

2. In the meantime, remove the heads of the anchovies, open them in two, down the center.,

3. rinse, and dry. Drain the endive, and put a third in a deep pyriform dish; cover with half of the anchovies, and dress with oil, the garlic, salt, and pepper.

4. Make the second layer of endive, and top with the rest of the anchovies.

5. Then dress in the same way with the remaining salad. Cook in the oven at 250°C for 45 to 50 minutes.

6. Serve warm, after sprinkling minced parsley over the dish.

Linguine With Fava Bean Pesto

4 servings

Ingredients

- 4 00g linguine
- 4 00 g fresh fava beans (shelled)
- 2 garlic clove
- Fresh mint
- 1 cup of extra virgin olive oil

Directions

1. Remove the skin of the fava beans., Then prepare the pesto by mashing the fava beans with the garlic a few mint leaves, and a bit of oil.

2. Cook the linguine in boiling water and drain when al dente, keeping some of the cooking water to dilute the sauce if too thick.

3. Toss the pasta with the pesto sauce, and serve.

Chocolate Almond Delights

Ingredients

- 600g of dark chocolate
- 600g of shelled almonds, unpeeled

Directions

1. Toast the almonds. Melt the chocolate in a bagno maria; add the almonds; mix.

2. Using a spoon, divide the mixture into 40 ramekin dishes.

3. Let cool until the chocolate is solidified.

Pasta And Beans

Serves 4

Ingredients

- 2 Fresh Onion

- 600g fresh Lamon beans or 600g of dried beans

- Kosher salt

- 10-15 Cloves

- 400g of tagliolini egg pasta or ditalini pasta

Directions

1. It is recommended to cook the beans in a pressure pot.

2. Fill the po pot until it reaches the level indicator.

3. Add a small handful of the kosher salt.

4. Cook on the highest flame; when the pressure pot whistles, lower the flame to the minimum, and cook for 45 to 50 minutes.

5. Puree the beans with a vegetable mill or hand blender, and pour into a large pot.

6. Easily bring to a boil, and add the fresh Onion and approx. 2 liter of water.

7. When the water reaches a boil, add the pasta; remove from the the heat; stir periodically so that the pasta does not stick.

8. The pasta and beans can be served hot or warm.

9. A nice addition is Treviso red radicchio, chopped into pieces.

10. The bitter flavor aids liver and kidney function during digestion.

11. Or it is possible to add a tablespoon of trippe alla parmigiana, which increases the protein content of the dish.

12. Finally, drizzle extra virgin olive oil over the finished dish— as should be done with all the dishes.

13. Then sprinkle some pepper over the dish, as pepper stimulates digestive secretion.

14. To finish the plate, add a pinch of Franco's "magic powder" dried sage, rosemary, thyme, and marjoram.

Berry Smoothie

Ingredients:

- 10 almonds (chopped)
- ¾ cup fat free Greek yogurt
- 2 cup strawberries (sliced)
- ¾ cup blueberries

Directions:

1. Place everything into your prepared blender together and let them blend until well combined.

2. Once the mixture is combined, you can pour it out into a glass and serve the drink right away.

Spiced Oatmeal

Ingredients:

- 25 to 30 scoops zone protein powder

- 2 6 Pecans (halves)

- 2 tsp pumpkin spice

- 2 tsp Stevia Extract

- ¾ cup Oats (steel cut)

- 2 cup apple sauce

- 4 cups water

Directions:

1. Pour the water in a large sauce pan and easily bring it to boil.

2. Next add in the oats and pumpkin spice and simply allow it to cook for approximately 5 to 10 minutes over high heat.

3. Lower the heat and simply allow the oats to simmer for approximately 45 to 50 minutes.

4. Now stir in the protein powder along with the rest of the ingredients and cook for another ten minutes or so.

Bacon Omelet With Fruits

Ingredients:

- 4 cup strawberries

- 2 fresh Onion (diced)

- 2 tbsp milk (2 %)

- Cooking spray

- 4 bacon slices

- 2 egg (whole)

- 2 tbsp green bell peppers

- 2 kiwi

Directions:

1. Spray some cooking spray in a small skillet.

2. Throw in the fresh Onions and pepper and simply allow it to cook on medium heat.

3. In a mixing bowl, whisk together the eggs with the milk.

4. Add the mixture to the skillet along with the diced bacon.

5. Gently simply allow the omelet to cook for 50 seconds or so before flipping it.

6. Transfer the omelet on to a plate and enjoy it with fresh fruits.

Egg Veggies

Ingredients:

- 2 tbsp vegetable stock (unsalted)

- 1/2 cup chives (chopped)

- 1/2 cup cream cheese (dairy free)

- 4 tbsp almond milk (unsweetened, divided)

- 2 fresh orange

- 2 tbsp salt

- 2 tsp olive oil (extra virgin)

- 4 cup egg whites (beaten)

- 1 cup ham (chopped)

- 6 tomatoes (peeled and chopped)

- 1 cup fresh Onion (finely chopped)

- 2 cup spinach (chopped)

Directions:

1. Preheat the oven to 450 degrees F,

2. Spray two oven friendly bowls with oil and set it aside.

3. In a small mixing bowl, mix the tomatoes with the salt and pour it equally among the three bowls.

4. In a skillet combine the vegetable stock with fresh Onions and oil.

5. Cook over medium heat for approximately 5 to 10 minutes.

6. Add the ham to it and cook for another minute or so.

7. Remove from heat and mix in the spinach.

8. In another mixing bowl, whisk together the egg with cream cheese, milk and chives.

9. Pour the mixture equally into the two bowls.

10. Now add the ham and vegetable mixture to the bowls and simply allow it to bake for approximately 35 to 40 minutes.

11. Add some salt and pepper to taste.

12. Serve with fresh fresh orange on the side.

Barbecue Beef With Onions

Ingredients

- 1/7 tsp Cumin

- 1/7 tsp Oregano

- 2 cup Onion - in half rings

- 2 clove Garlic - minced

- 2 cup Mushrooms

- 2 tsps Kitchen Basics unsalted vegetable stock

- 2 tsp White wine vinegar

- 2 cup Snow peas

- 4 tsp Virgin Olive Oil - divided

- 4 oz Beef, eye of round

- 1 cup Tomato puree

- 2 tsp Worcestershire sauce

- 1/2 tsp Cider vinegar

- 1/2 tsp Chili powder

Instructions

1. In skillet add1 tsp oil and beef. Cook beef until no longer pink.

2. Add puree, Worcestershire sauce, cider vinegar, chili powder, cumin and oregano. Cover and simmer 6 minutes until sauce forms.

3. In another skillet add remaining oil, fresh Onion, and garlic and cook until onion is tender.

4. Add onion, garlic, mushrooms, beef stock, and white wine vinegar to beef. Cover and cook 8 minutes.

5. Add snow peas after 6 minutes.

6. Stir to blend flavors.

Baked Tilapia With Vegetables

Ingredients

- 1/2 cup Bell pepper - sliced, 2 medium

- 1/2 cup Tomato- sliced, 2 medium

- 1/2 cup Red onion - sliced, 2 medium

- Salt and pepper - to taste

- Herbs - to your liking

- 4 tsps Dr. Sears' Zone Extra virgin olive oil

- 1 cup Strawberries

- 4 oz Tilapia

- 4 cups Summer squash - sliced, 2 medium

- 4 cups Zucchini - sliced, 2 medium

Instructions:

1. Preheat oven to 4 60°F.

2. Place fish in cooking-oil-sprayed bakeware with sliced vegetables. Sprinkle salt and pepper.

3. Spray with olive oil.

4. Add fresh herbs of your choice.

5. Bake 25 to 30 minutes or until fish flakes.

6. Easily put on your plate and drizzle with extra virgin olive oil.

7. Have strawberries for dessert.

Baked Fusilli With Zucchini

Ingredients

- 2 slice Canadian Bacon (chopped to bite-sized pieces)

- Salt and pepper (to taste)

- 2 Tbsp Mozzarella Cheese (shredded, part-skim milk)

- 2 tsp Parmesan Cheese (grated)

- Cooking Spray

- 1 cup Zone PastaRx Fusilli

- 1 cup Zucchini - cut into small cubes

- 1 cup Green Beans (trimmed and cut diagonally in half)

- 2 tsp Olive Oil

- 1 (2 4 oz) can Diced Tomatoes

- 1 cup Tomato Sauce

- 2 Tbsp Water

- 1/2 tsp Italian Seasoning

Instructions:

1. Preheat oven to 450°F.

2. Prepare Zone PastaRx Fusilli according to package directions with zucchini and green beans.

3. Heat oil in skillet over medium-high heat.

4. Stir in olive oil, diced tomatoes with juice, fresh tomato sauce, 1-5 tablespoons of water, Italian

seasoning, Canadian bacon, salt and pepper. Cover and simmer for 4 minutes.

5. Transfer into small baking dish coated with cooking spray. Sprinkle with mozzarella and Parmesan cheeses.

6. Cover and bake for 25 to 30 minutes or until bubbly.

7. Uncover and bake for 6 minutes longer.

Baked Scallops

Ingredients

- 4 cups Romaine lettuce - chopped
- 1/2 cup Garbanzo beans - reduced sodium, bush's
- 2 Tomato
- 2 cup Cucumber
- 4 oz Bay scallops
- 4 tbsps White wine - for marinade
- 2 tbsp Rolled oats - old fashioned
- 1 oz Low-fat cheddar cheese - shredded
- 4 tsps Extra virgin olive oil
- 4 tbsps Fresh squeezed lemon juice

Instructions:

1. Marinate scallops in white cooking wine overnight in the refrigerator

2. Preheat oven to 460°F.

3. Drain scallops and place in an individual baking dish, sprinkle with old fashioned oats and then spread shredded cheese on top.

4. Bake for 25 to 30 minutes.

5. While the scallops are baking, whisk the extra virgin olive oil, fresh lemon juice and Mrs. Dash together for a dressing.

6. Combine garbanzo beans with the rest of the salad ingredients and drizzle with dressing.

Pork, Apples And Eggs

Ingredients:

- 2 boneless pork filets, about 2-ounces each
- Salt and pepper to taste
- 2 teaspoon olive oil

For the apples:

- 2 medium apple, cored and sliced
- 1/2 teaspoon cinnamon
- Complete the meal with:

- 1 cup beaten egg whites, scrambled

- 2 cup sliced strawberries

Instructions:

1. Heat the olive oil in a skillet to medium heat.

2. Season the pork chops with salt and pepper to taste; sprinkle the cinnamon over the apples.

3. Cook the pork on one side of the skillet and the apples on the other side for about 25 to 30 minutes or until pork is not pink and the apples are tender.

4. Remove from the skillet and serve with the remainder of the meal.

Mighty Minestrone Soup

Ingredients:

- 1/2 cup cooked black beans

- 1/2 cup cooked chickpeas

- 1/2 cup dry elbow macaroni

- 2 teaspoons olive oil

- 2 minced cloves of garlic

- 4 cups low-fat beef broth

- 2 teaspoon each: dried basil and oregano

- Salt and pepper to taste

- 8 ounces of lean, cubed beef

- 2 stalks celery, diced

- 2 medium fresh Onion, diced

- 2 cups shredded cabbage

- 1 cup crushed tomatoes

Instructions:

1. In a pot, combine everything but the dry macaroni noodles; cook for 25 to 30 minutes or until the vegetables are tender.

2. Add the macaroni to the soup and cook for another 25 to 30 minutes or until the macaroni is done to taste.

Surprise Meatball Soup

!

Ingredients:

- 2 teaspoon grated ginger

- 2 teaspoon chopped parsley

- 1 teaspoon hot sauce, or to taste

- 25 ounces chicken, ground

- 1 small fresh Onion, finely diced

For the soup:

- 1/2 cup cornstarch mixed with1 cup water

- 2 teaspoons virgin olive oil

- Salt and pepper to taste

- Complete the meal with:

- 1 cup unsweetened applesauce

- 4 cups low-fat and low-sodium chicken broth

- 2 additional small fresh Onion, cut into rings

- 2 cups sliced leeks

- 8 ounces sliced mushrooms

Instructions:

1. Preheat the oven to 450 degrees. Lightly spray a baking sheet with oil.

2. Make the meatballs: Combine the meatball ingredients and form into small, bite-sized balls.

3. Bake for 35 to 40 minutes or until done.

4. Place the soup ingredients in a saucepan and easily bring to a rolling boil; lower the heat and cook until vegetables are tender, about 35 to 40 minutes.

5. Add1 of the cornstarch mixture to the vegetable pot and cook for 2 minute or until thickened; add more of the cornstarch as really needed until the desired thickness is reached. If the soup becomes too thick, add water.

6. When the meatballs are done, add them to the soup mixture and cook an additional minute to blend the flavors.

Bean Stew Mexican Style

Ingredients:

- 1 cup prepared salsa, mild or to taste

- 4 teaspoons olive oil

- 1/2 cup water

- 2 tablespoons chopped cilantro

- 2 teaspoon lime zest

- 8 ounces chicken breasts, diced

- 2 cup black beans or pintos, drained and rinsed, if canned

- 1 cup chopped fresh Onion

- 1/2 cup chopped zucchini

- 2 cup crushed tomatoes

- Salt and pepper to taste

Instructions:

1. Heat the olive oil to medium in a saucepan.

2. Add the beans, zucchini and fresh Onion; cook for 5 to 10 minutes or until fresh Onion is tender.

3. Remove to another saucepan.

4. Brown the chicken in the same olive oil coated pan for 5 to 10 minutes; add to the zucchini mixture in the other saucepan.

5. Add the remaining ingredients to the chicken/zucchini pot and cook for another 25 to 30 minutes or until vegetables are done completely.

Perfect Veal Goulash

Ingredients:

- 6 cloves of garlic, minced (or to taste)

- 2 cups low-fat beef stock

- 1/2 teaspoon caraway seed

- 2 tablespoons smoked paprika, or to taste

- 2 tablespoon Worcestershire sauce, or to taste

- Pepper to taste

- 2 tablespoon cornstarch mixed with1/2 cup water

- 2 tablespoon fresh basil, chopped

- 4 teaspoons olive oil

- 8 ounces choice veal, cubed to 4 inch pieces

- 4 cups diced fresh Onion

- 2 cups fresh tomato puree or crushed tomatoes

Instructions:

1. Preheat the oven to 450 degrees.

2. Coat the bottom of a 2 quart casserole dish with the olive oil.

3. Combine all the ingredients, except the cornstarch mixture and the basil, in a bowl and stir together well; transfer the mixture to the coated casserole dish.

4. Cover the dish tightly with foil and cook for 25 to 30 minutes in the oven.

5. Remove the casserole from the oven; add the cornstarch mixture and the basil. Stir well; return the casserole to the hot oven and cook another 25 to 30 minutes, covered tightly.

Cauliflower Mash

- 30 tablespoons yogurt, Greek variety is best, plain

- 2 teaspoon virgin olive oil

- 8 ounces frozen cauliflower

- 2 tablespoons low-sodium chicken stock

- Salt and pepper to taste

1. Cook the cauliflower until tender; mash well.

2. Add the remaining ingredients and stir to combine completely

Mustard Drizzle Dressing

Ingredients

- 2 tablespoon white wine vinegar

- 2 teaspoons honey

- 2 tablespoon Dijon mustard

- 4 tablespoons extra-virgin olive oil

- Salt and pepper (optional)

DIRECTIONS

1. Heat oven to 450 degrees.

2. In a large mixing bowl, toss potatoes with garlic, herbs, and half of olive oil.

3. Place in a single layer in a roasting pan and roast for 30 to 35 minutes, stirring once or twice.

4. When potatoes are tender and starting to brown, add the chickpeas and green beans and roast for another 25 to 30 minutes.

5. While that roasts, in a small bowl whisk together mustard, olive oil, vinegar, and honey to form an emulsified dressing.

6. Season the dressing with salt and pepper to taste.

7. Transfer the roasted vegetables and beans to a platter and drizzle with dressing. Serve warm.

Ikarian Stuffed Eggplant

INGREDIENTS

- 2 onions, diced

- 4 cloves garlic, sliced in thirds

- 2 cup extra-virgin olive oil

- 2 potato, peeled and thinly sliced

- 2 bell pepper (green, red, or yellow), diced

- 6 medium eggplants, ends cut off, scored deeply four times lengthwise

- 2 cup parsley, chopped

- 2 large tomatoes, diced

- Salt and pepper to taste

Directions:

1. In a large pan, sauté eggplants in olive oil for about 25 to 30 minutes, rotating often.

2. In a medium bowl, mix together parsley, tomatoes, onions, garlic, bell pepper, and 4 cup olive oil as your stuffing mixture.

3. In a separate pan, sauté stuffing for 10 to 15 minutes, or until onions are tender.

4. Add the stuffing mix on top and into the eggplants.

5. Place potatoes around the eggplants in the pan.

6. Cook over low heat for about 45 to 50 minutes, checking the pan for liquid

and basting with cooking liquid, if really needed.

Instant Pot One-Pot Pasta With Cherry Tomatoes And Basil

Ingredients

- 5-10 cups water

- 2 pint (6 62 ml) cherry tomatoes

- 2 bunch fresh basil, torn or sliced

- 1/2 cup drained capers

- 2 cup shredded vegan Parmesan cheese

- 2 small yellow onion, diced

- 8 cloves garlic, sliced

- 1/2 teaspoon red pepper flakes

- 2 lb (4 60g) uncooked short pasta (such as penne, fusilli, or bowtie)

- 2 teaspoon sea salt

- Freshly ground

DIRECTIONS

1. On the Instant Pot, select Sauté and heat the oil, if using, in the inner pot until hot.

2. Add the onion and sauté until softened and golden, 5 to 10 minutes.

3. Add the garlic and pepper and sauté 2 minute longer.

4. Add the pasta to the inner pot of the Instant Pot.

5. Add the salt and water until just covered, no more than 1/2 inch (0.

6cm) above the pasta. Add the tomatoes on top without stirring.

6. Lock the lid of the Instant Pot and ensure the steam release valve is set to the sealing position.

7. Select Pressure Cook (Low), and set the cook time for half of the cook time on the pasta package, rounding down.

8. For example, if the pasta package calls for 25 to 30 to 25 minutes on the stove, set the cook time for 5 to 10 minutes.

9. Once the cook time is complete, immediately quick release the pressure and carefully remove the lid.

10. Add the fresh basil and capers, and stir to combine.

11. Drizzle with a little olive oil, if desired.

12.   Serve immediately with Parmesan and salt and pepper, to taste.

Pantry-Style Spicy Street Noodles

INGREDIENTS

- 2 tablespoon vegetable oil

- 2 small sweet onion, thinly sliced into strips

- 8 oz firm tofu, cut into strips (optional)

- 2 teaspoons minced garlic

- 2-4 cups chopped greens (spinach, bok choy, kale, mustard greens, shredded cabbage, green beans, or any combination of these)

- 25 oz fettuccine or rice noodles

- 2 teaspoon ground cumin

- 2-4 teaspoon sambal oelek or other sweet chili sauce like sriracha

- 4 tablespoons ketchup

- 2 tablespoons soy sauce

- Lemon for serving

Directions:

1. Cook noodles according to package directions. Drain well.

2. Heat up a large pan or wok over high heat.

3. Add the oil, reduce heat to medium-high and saute the onion for 2-4 minutes.

4. Add garlic, greens, and tofu, if using, to pan and cook for another 4 minutes.

5. Mix spice and sauces in a bowl.

6. Add noodles to the pan, tossing and mixing with tongs or cooking chopsticks.

7. Add spice – sauce mixture and toss everything together.

8. Cook for another 5-10 minutes, until everything is combined and seasoned.

9. Transfer to individual serving bowls and serve with lemon wedges and sambal oelek.

French Lentils With Roasted Radishes

INGREDIENTS

- 4 large cloves garlic, pressed

- 2 tablespoons minced fresh mint

- 1/2 cup minced fresh chives

- 4 tablespoons hemp seeds, divided

- 2 tablespoons fresh lemon juice

- 2 cups (packed) mâché or baby spinach

- 1 cup almond ricotta

- 4 cups Puy (French) lentils, or black lentils

- 2 bay leaf

- Sea salt and ground black pepper

- 4 cups radishes

- 4 tablespoons olive oil, divided

Directions:

1. Preheat the oven to 4 60°F.

2. In a medium saucepan over high heat, combine the lentils and the bay leaf with about 6 cups of water.

3. Easily bring to a boil, and then reduce the heat to medium-low.

4. Simmer gently until the lentils are tender but not mushy, about 30 to 35 minutes.

5. Drain the lentils in a colander over the sink, and remove the bay leaf.

6. Transfer the lentils to a bowl and season them with 1 teaspoon salt and 1 teaspoon ground black pepper. Cover the bowl to keep the lentils warm.

7. Meanwhile, clean and trim the radishes, removing the stems, while leaving their tails intact.Halve the radishes lengthwise, and quarter any large halves.

8. Warm 2 tablespoon of the olive oil in an ovenproof saute pan over medium-high heat.

9. When the oil is hot, add the radishes to the pan in a single layer season generously with salt and pepper, and cook for 5-10 minutes to lightly sear the bottoms.

10. Remove the pan from the heat, stir in the garlic, distributing it well, and transfer the pan to the oven.

11. Roast the radishes for 8 –25 minutes until they are vibrantly red and lightly golden on the edges. Remove the pan from the oven.

12. In a large mixing bowl, combine the cooked lentils, roasted radishes and their cooking juices, and the remaining 2 tablespoons of olive oil.

13. Add the mint, chives, 2 tablespoons of the hemp seeds, lemon juice, and the mache or baby spinach to the bowl.

14. Toss the mixture to combine and season to taste with additional salt and pepper as desired.

15. Add the almond ricotta to the mixture in small dollops and fold it into the mixture gently, retaining the dollops as much as possible.

16. Sprinkle the remaining tablespoon of hemp seeds on top, and serve warm or at room temperature.

Blueberry Chia Muffins

Ingredients:

- ¾ cup almond milk
- 8 tablespoons maple syrup
- 2 teaspoon vanilla extract
- 2 cup frozen blueberries
- 4 cup spelt flour
- 2 tablespoon baking powder
- 1 teaspoon sea salt
- ¾ teaspoon cinnamon
- 1 teaspoon cardamom
- 4 tablespoons chia seeds
- 6 tablespoons coconut oil

DIRECTIONS

1. Whisk dry ingredients.

2. Melt coconut oil on stovetop, mix in other wet ingredients over gentle heat until smooth.

3. Mix wet ingredients into dry ingredients.

4. Carefully stir in blueberries.

5. Scoop into muffin tin.

6. Sprinkle remaining chia seeds on top of muffins.

7. Bake in oven at 450 degrees F for 35 to 40 minutes.

Strawberry Lemonade Breakfast Soft-Serve

Ingredients:

2 tablespoons maple syrup

Nondairy milk, as needed to blend

Optional Toppings

2 frozen bananas

2 cups frozen strawberries

Juice of 2 fresh lemon

Additional banana and strawberry slices

Fruit

Granola

Cacao nibs

Dollop of nut butter

Chia seeds

Nuts

Unsweetened shredded coconut

Directions

1. To prepare the soft serve, add the bananas, strawberries, fresh lemon juice, maple syrup, and 2 tablespoon of nondairy milk to a blender or food processor.

2. Blend, adding 2 tablespoon of milk at a time, as needed, until a texture similar to that of soft-serve is formed.

3. Transfer the ice cream to bowls, add your choice of toppings, and enjoy right away.

4. Keep a stash of bananas in the freezer so you can have soft-serve in a flash.

5. The easiest way to freeze and store bananas is to peel them and slice them into 2 -inch pieces.

6. Then place the pieces on a baking sheet lined with parchment paper, freeze them for 2-2 ½ hours, and transfer them to an airtight container and store in the freezer until needed.

Instant Pot One-Pot Pasta With Cherry Tomatoes And Basil

Ingredients

4– 6 cups water

2 pint (6 62 ml) cherry tomatoes

2 bunch fresh basil, torn or sliced

1/2 cup drained capers

2 cup shredded vegan Parmesan cheese

Freshly ground

2 small yellow fresh Onion, diced

4 cloves garlic, sliced

1/2 teaspoon red pepper flakes

2 lb (4 60g) uncooked short pasta (such as penne, fusilli, or bowtie)

2 teaspoon sea salt

Directions

1. On the Instant Pot, select Sauté and heat the oil, if using, in the inner pot until hot.

2. Add the onion and sauté until softened and golden, 5 to 10 minutes.

3. Add the garlic and pepper and sauté 2 minute longer.

4. Press Cancel.

5. Add the pasta to the inner pot of the Instant Pot.

6. Add the salt and water until just covered, no more than 1/2 inch (0. 6cm) above the pasta.

7. Add the tomatoes on top without stirring.

8. Lock the lid of the Instant Pot and ensure the steam release valve is set to the sealing position.

9. Select Pressure Cook (Low), and set the cook time for half of the cook time on the pasta package, rounding down. For example, if the pasta package calls for 40 to 45 minutes on the stove, set the cook time for 5 to 10 minutes.

10. Once the cook time is complete, immediately quick release the pressure and carefully remove the lid.

11. Add the fresh basil and capers, and stir to combine.

12. Drizzle with a little olive oil, if desired.

13.   Serve immediately with Parmesan and salt and pepper, to taste.

Pantry-Style Spicy Street Noodles (Mee Goreng)

Ingredients

- 2 teaspoon ground cumin

- 2-4 teaspoon sambal oelek or other sweet chili sauce like sriracha

- 4 tablespoons ketchup

- 2 tablespoons soy sauce

- Lemon for serving

- 2 tablespoon vegetable oil

- 2 small sweet fresh Onion, thinly sliced into strips

- 2 teaspoons minced garlic

- 2-4 cups chopped greens

- 25 oz fettuccine or rice noodles

Directions

1. Cook noodles according to package directions.

2. Drain well. Heat up a large pan or wok over high heat.

3. Add the oil, reduce heat to medium-high and saute the onion for 5-10   minutes.

4. Add garlic, greens, and tofu, if using, to pan and cook for another 5 to 10 minutes.

5. Mix spice and sauces in a bowl.

6. Add noodles to the pan, tossing and mixing with tongs or cooking chopsticks.

7. Add spice – sauce mixture and toss everything together.

8. Cook for another 2-4 minutes, until everything is combined and seasoned.

9. Transfer to individual serving bowls and serve with fresh lemon wedges and sambal oelek.

French Lentils With Roasted Radishes

INGREDIENTS

- 4 tablespoons olive oil, divided

- 4 large cloves garlic, pressed

- 2 tablespoons minced fresh mint

- 1/2 cup minced fresh chives

- 4 tablespoons hemp seeds, divided

- 2 tablespoons fresh fresh lemon juice

- 2 cups (packed) mâché or baby spinach

- 1 cup almond ricotta

- 4 cups Puy (French) lentils, or black lentils

- 2 bay leaf

- Sea salt and ground black pepper

- 4 cups radishes

Directions:

1. Preheat the oven to 4 60°F.

2. In a medium saucepan over high heat, combine the lentils and the bay leaf with about 10 cups of water.

3. Easily bring to a boil, and then reduce the heat to medium-low.

4. Simmer gently until the lentils are tender but not mushy, about 25-30 minutes.

5. Drain the lentils in a colander over the sink, and remove the bay leaf.

6. Transfer the lentils to a bowl and season them with 1 teaspoon salt and 1 teaspoon ground black pepper.

7. Cover the bowl to keep the lentils warm.

8. Meanwhile, clean and trim the radishes, removing the stems, while leaving their tails intact.

9. Halve the radishes lengthwise, and quarter any large halves.

10. Warm 2 tablespoon of the olive oil in an ovenproof saute pan* over medium-high heat.

11. When the oil is hot, add the radishes to the pan in a single layer season generously with salt and pepper, and cook for 5-10 minutes to lightly sear the bottoms.

12. Remove the pan from the heat, stir in the garlic, distributing it well, and

transfer the pan to the oven. Roast the radishes for 25-30 minutes until they are vibrantly red and lightly golden on the edges.

13.   Remove the pan from the oven.

14.   In a large mixing bowl, combine the cooked lentils, roasted radishes and their cooking juices, and the remaining 2 tablespoons of olive oil. Add the mint, chives, 2 tablespoons of the hemp seeds, fresh lemon juice, and the mache or baby spinach to the bowl.

15.   Toss the mixture to combine and season to taste with additional salt and pepper as desired.

16.   Add the almond ricotta to the mixture in small dollops and fold it into the mixture gently, retaining the dollops as much as possible.

17. Sprinkle the remaining tablespoon of hemp seeds on top, and serve warm or at room temperature.

Blueberry Chia Muffins

Ingredients

- 8 tablespoons maple syrup
- 2 teaspoon vanilla extract
- 2 cup frozen blueberries
- 4 cup spelt flour
- 2 tablespoon baking powder
- 1 teaspoon sea salt
- ¾ teaspoon cinnamon
- 1 teaspoon cardamom
- 4 tablespoons chia seeds
- 6 tablespoons coconut oil

- ¾ cup almond milk (oat milk, coconut milk, etc.)

Directions:

1. Whisk dry ingredients. Melt coconut oil on stovetop, mix in other wet ingredients over gentle heat until smooth.

2. Mix wet ingredients into dry ingredients.

3. Carefully stir in blueberries. Scoop into muffin tin.

4. Sprinkle remaining chia seeds on top of muffins.

5. Bake in oven at 450 degrees F for 45-50 minutes.

Instant Pot Quinoa Breakfast Bowls

Ingredients

- 2 cup quinoa, rinsed and drained
- 4 cups unsweetened almond or other plant-based milk, plus more to serve
- 1 teaspoon pure vanilla extract
- Pinch of ground cinnamon

FOR SERVING INGREDIENTS

- 2 cup berries
- 2 banana, sliced

- 1/2 cup pure maple syrup

Directions:

1. In the inner pot, stir together the quinoa, almond milk, vanilla, and cinnamon.

2. Lock the lid and ensure the steam release valve is set to the sealing position.

3. Select Pressure Cook and set the cook time for 5 to 10 minutes.

4. Once the cook time is complete, immediately quick release the pressure.

5. Carefully remove the lid. If desired, stir in more milk to thin into a porridge.

6. Serve warm in bowls, sweetened to taste with maple syrup and topped generously with fruit and almonds.

1 cup slivered almonds, toasted

Strawberry Lemonade Breakfast Soft-Serve

INGREDIENTS

- Juice of 2 lemon

- 2 tablespoons maple syrup

- Nondairy milk, as needed to blend

- Optional Toppings

- Granola

- Nuts

- Unsweetened shredded coconut

- Cacao nibs

- Dollop of nut butter

- 2 frozen bananas

- 2 cups frozen strawberries

- Additional banana and strawberry slices

- Fruit

- Chia seeds

Directions:

1. To prepare the soft serve, add the bananas, strawberries, fresh lemon juice, maple syrup, and 2 tablespoon of nondairy milk to a blender or food processor.

2. Blend, adding 2 tablespoon of milk at a time, as needed, until a texture similar to that of soft-serve is formed.

3. Transfer the ice cream to bowls, add your choice of toppings, and enjoy right away.

Break Free Breakfast Burrito With Grapefruit

INGREDIENTS:

- 1 med Grapefruit
- 2 Tbsp   Salsa
- 2   Tortillas, flour, 6 inch
- fl   oz   Cheese,   monterey   jack,   2%, shredded
- 4 Egg Whites
- Egg, whole

DIRECTIONS:

1. Warm tortilla in microwave or frying pan.

2. Scramble eggs, seasoned to taste, and place on tortilla. top with salsa and cheese.

3. Roll up and serve with grapefruit.

Mesmerizing Melon Smoothie

An exotic and summery smoothie!

INGREDIENTS:

- 4 scoop of protein powder

- 2 Cup of Strawberries

- 1/2 Cups of Water

- 2 Cup of Melon

- 4 Tbsp Nuts

- 1/2 Cup of canned peaches

DIRECTIONS:

1. Rinse peaches, remove stems from strawberries.

2. Cube cantaloupe.

3. Mix all ingredients in blender until smooth

Kickstart Your Day Kale Smoothie

A supremely energizing green smoothie!

INGREDIENTS:

- banana (broken into chunks)
- 1/2 cup frozen blueberries
- scoops Protein Powder
- 2 tsp extra virgin olive oil
- 4 cups kale (rib cut from leaf, chopped)
- 4 cups water ((desired consistency) add ice or decrease water amount)
- avocado (scooped from skin, chopped)

DIRECTIONS:

1. Blend kale and water in blender.

2. Add avocado and banana; blend again.

3. Add berries and Protein Powder. Blend until smooth.

4. Blend until you have the consistency you want.

5. Add the extra virgin olive oil at the end and pulse a few times.

Mexican Omelette

INGREDIENTS:

- cup green bell pepper - diced
- 1 cup red bell pepper - diced
- cup mushrooms - minced
- cups Egg whites
- 1/7 tsp black pepper
- 1/2 tsp hot sauce
- 1/7 tsp dry mustard
- 1/2 tsp turmeric
- 1/7 tsp chili powder
- 6 tsp olive oil - divided
- 4 cups fresh Onions - minced
- 4 cloves garlic - pressed, divided
- 1/2 cup garbanzo beans canned
- cup black beans canned

Directions:

1. Firstly, In a medium sauté pan heat 4 teaspoon olive oil to medium heat.

2. Cook the fresh Onion, garlic, garbanzo beans, black beans, peppers and mushrooms until they are tender.

3. In a mixing bowl, whisk together 4 teaspoons olive oil, egg whites, black pepper, hot sauce, mustard, turmeric, and chili powder.

4. Then in a second sauté pan, a large one, heat 4 teaspoons oil and spread it around the whole pan before adding the egg mixture. C

5. cook until set, and an omelet is formed.

6. Fill omelet with the vegetable mixture, fold over, cut in half and serve.

OH SO TASTY OKRA BREAKFAST

INGREDIENTS:

2 tbsp Jalapeño Peppers - Canned

1/2 cup Okra - Fresh/Tender - Thinly Sliced

2 tbsp Fresh tomato Sauce

1 cup Water - Do Not Add All at Once

1 cup Egg Whites

Salt and Pepper - To Taste

1 cup Blueberries

2 Clove Garlic - Chopped

2 tbsp Sweet Fresh Onion - Chopped

2 link Al Fresco Sweet Apple Chicken Sausage

1 tsp Olive Oil

1 cup Chopped Tomato

DIRECTIONS:

1. Sauté garlic, fresh Onion and chicken sausage in olive oil over medium heat for approximately 5 to 10 minutes.

2. Add chopped fresh tomato and jalapeños and sauté for 5 to 10 minutes or until veggies are tender.

3. Add okra and sauté for another minute.

4. Add fresh tomato sauce and about ½ cup water.

5. Stir to make a sauce.

6. Add egg and let set before mixing.

7. Add more water if you want more of a saucy constancy.

8. Finish with blueberries.

Superb Slow Poached Pears
With Very Vanilla Sauce

INGREDIENTS:

- 4 1 cups 0%-Fat Greek Yogurt
- 2 tbsp Extra Virgin Olive Oil
- 2 tsp Pure Vanilla Extract
- 4 scoops   Protein Powder
- 1/7 tsp Stevia - to taste
- 2 6 Macadamia Nuts - chopped
- 4   Pears - small ripe but not mushy
- 1/2 cup Grapes - halved
- 1/2 cup Blueberries

- 1/2 cup Water

- 2 tsp Grated Fresh lemon - or fresh orange rind or 1/2 teaspoon dried

- 4 tsp Ginger Root - or Hawaii Naturals bottled ginger puree

- 2 Cinnamon Stick

Directions:

1. Remove core from bottom of pears with apple corer while leaving stem intact.

2. Peel and arrange in 21 to 4 2 /2- quart slow cooker.

3. Sprinkle with grape halves and blueberries.

4. Combine water, fresh lemon or fresh orange rind, and ginger, then pour over pears.

5. Easily put cinnamon stick in the middle of the cooker. Cover and cook on LOW for 21 to 4 hours, until fork tender.

6. Combine yogurt, extra virgin olive oil, vanilla and stevia. Stir and taste. Add more stevia if a sweeter taste is desired.

7. When pears are cooked, cut in quarters from the top down and divide between 4 serving bowls.

8. Evenly distribute cooking juices and remaining fruit among serving bowls.

9. Top the fruit with yogurt mix and sprinkle with nuts.

Magnificent Museli

- 4 walnuts - coarsely chopped

- 4   Macadamia   Nuts   -   coarsely chopped

- 4 scoops Protein Powder

- 2 cups 0%-Fat Greek yogurt

- 2   Apple - small, cored and grated

- 2   Pear - small, cored and grated or 1/2 of a ripe banana, sliced

- 2 cup Steel Cut Oats

- 2 tbsp Dried Cranberries

- 2   Dried   Apricots - 4   sulfite-free whole or 6 halves, minced

- 2 tsp Apple Pie Spice - or cinnamon

- 25 Almonds - coarsely chopped

- 8 Pecan Halves - coarsely chopped

Directions:

1. Lightly toast oats and nut pieces in a dry skillet over medium-low heat, stirring all the while, until lightly golden and aromatic, 10-15 minutes.

2. Toss oats, nuts, dried fruits, spice, and protein powder in medium bowl.

3. Before going to bed, add yogurt to oat-nut mixture.

4. Stir, cover and refrigerate overnight.

5. In the morning, wash, core, and grate fresh fruit.

6. Add to muesli, stir, then let stand for 35 to 40 minutes.

7. If desired, add a bit more water. Divide among 5 cereal bowls and serve.

Appletastic Wonderful Walnut Chicken Pastsa

INGREDIENTS:

- link Al fresco sweet apple chicken sausage - sliced

- 1/2 medium apple - diced

- 1/2 tsp walnuts - crushed, toasted if you want

- cup baby spinach leaves

- 1/2 cup pasta

- 1 tsp olive oil

- tbsp dry white cooking wine

- 2 slice fresh Onion

124

Directions:

1. Cook Pasta as directed on packet.

2. Drain. Reserve1 cup of liquid and set aside.

3. Heat oil and wine in nonstick skillet.

4. Sauté fresh Onion until translucent, about 5-10 minutes.

5. Add cut sausage and cook until heated through, about 1-5 minutes.

6. Stir in diced apples, walnuts, spinach and reserved pasta.

7. Add some of the reserved water if needed.

8. Cook for an additional 2 minutes until all ingredients are warm and spinach is wilted.

Awesome Applesauce Burgers
With Superfood Spinach

INGREDIENTS:

2 tsp Water

2 tsp Polaner sugar free All Fruit - or flavor of your choice

Salt and pepper - to taste

4 cups Baby spinach - tear stems off

2 slices Red fresh Onion - roughly chopped

1 Fresh tomato - cut

1 cup Strawberries - cut into chunks

1/2 cup Unsweetened applesauce

4 tbsp   oats

2 tsp dehydrated fresh Onion flakes - to taste

1 tsp chili powder

4 oz Ground chicken breast

Dressing & Spinach Salad

4 tsp Olive oil

2 tsp Vinegar

DIRECTIONS:

1. Firstly, preheat the broiler.

2. Next, in a bowl, mix together ½ cup applesauce, oatmeal, egg whites and fresh Onions.

3. Add the turkey.

4. Mix well and shape into a burger.

5. Spray non-heated broiler pan with nonstick coating.

6. Easily put burger on the rack.

7. You are going to want to broil it for five minutes and then turn it over. Broil five minutes more or until meat is no longer pink.

8. Heat remaining applesauce and serve over burger.

9. While the burger is cooking, whisk dressing ingredients together with a few mashed strawberries.

10. Mix spinach, fresh Onion, fresh tomato and strawberries in a salad bowl and drizzle with dressing.